Dedicatie

I would like to dedicate this book to all those people in the world who suffer from this terrible embarrassing illness called "Crohn's Disease"

Acknowledgements

I would like to thank the following people who have supported me through my life with Crohn's;

- My family, parents Bernard and Mary and brother Simon Judge.
- Jason's family, parents Stan and Yvonne, brother Brett and wife Leone, brother Adam Wright.
- Paul and Joan Phillips
- To all my wonderful friends, you know who you are. Thank you for your continual support and friendships.
- All those Doctors and nurses that have treated me over the years both in Australia and England.
- Alex Cannon for the photos used in this book.
- A special thank you to Belinda McCracken for giving me the idea to write this book.

To my wonderful son Daniel, you always put a smile on my face and I thank you from the bottom of my heart for your patience, caring and understanding as you were growing up. You make me so proud, I love you very much.

Finally, my husband Jason, you are my world, my rock and without you I don't think I would have found the strength to get through my life so far. No matter what happens, you are always there with a positive smile and attitude. Thank you for your continued love and support and for being the best husband and father in the world.
I LOVE YOU xxx

My Life with Crohn's Disease

Melanie Wright

Published 2008 by arima publishing

www.arimapublishing.com

ISBN 978 1 84549 342 4

Printed and bound in the United Kingdom

Typeset in Palatino Linotype 14/16

Swirl is an imprint of arima publishing.

arima publishing
ASK House, Northgate Avenue
Bury St Edmunds, Suffolk IP32 6BB
t: (+44) 01284 700321

www.arimapublishing.com

Contents

Introduction

My name is Melanie Wright, I'm 40 years young married to my husband Jason and we have an 18 year old son named Daniel. I was born in England 29th March 1968 and emigrated to Australia at the age of four with my parents Bernard and Mary and my older brother Simon Judge. Here we lived in a place called Emu Plains which is a suburb in Sydney until the age of 12. Then we moved to Nelson Bay which is in New South Wales where I completed my high school education. At the age of 16 my family moved us to Canberra, which is the capital of Australia where I met my husband Jason. We were married May 1988 and lived there for a further 10 years before we relocated to Manchester England in December of 1998 where we still reside today.

I am a hairdresser by profession, but unable to work due to my illness and have been suffering with Crohn's disease since October 1994. I wanted to write this book in order to help other Crohn's sufferers and their families to better understand how this disease can affect people in their everyday lives. Of course everyone's story and circumstances are different, however I hope that my story will not only enlighten, but give hope to others who have just been diagnosed with this terrible disease. To date there are hundreds of thousands of people living around the world who suffer from Crohn's.

This book is my way of bringing this disease to the publics attention in hope of better research and public understanding of what a Crohn's sufferer goes through on an every day basis. Crohn's is also known as an "embarrassing illness". When I was first diagnosed I found it very difficult to find information apart from a medical perspective. I really needed to find information from people who were living with the disease to help me both understand and prepare for what might lie ahead for me and my family.

Crohn's Disease is: A chronic inflammatory disease, primarily involving the small and large intestine, but which can affect other parts of the digestive system as well. It is named after Burrill Crohn, the American gastroenterologist who first described the disease in 1932.The most common part of the small intestine to be affected by Crohn's disease is the last portion, called the ileum. Active disease in this area is termed Crohn's ileitis. When both the small intestine and the large intestine are involved, the condition is called Crohn's enterocolitis (or ileocolitis). Abdominal pain, diarrhoea, vomiting, fever and weight loss are common symptoms. Crohn's disease can be associated with reddish tender skin nodules, and inflammation of the joints, spine, eyes, and liver. Diagnosis is commonly made by x-ray or colonoscopy. Treatment includes medications that are anti-inflammatory, immune suppressors or antibiotics. Surgery can be necessary in severe cases.

(a)

(b)

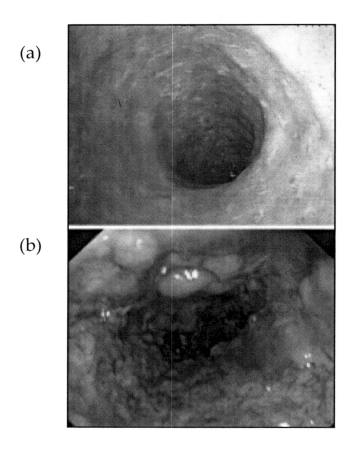

Photograph (a) shows a "healthy" bowel.

Photograph (b) shows a "diseased" bowel affected by Crohn's Disease.

Chapter One – Crohn's Diagnosis

Around the start of 1994, I started to feel unwell within myself. I noticed that I started to become constipated and found it very difficult to pass any bowel motion. I then started to notice blood appearing at this time and would find myself sitting on the toilet for very long periods of time and nothing happening. At night I was getting cramps in my calves and toes and mouth ulcers were becoming very common. I just ignored all of this and thought it would get better and simply go away.

As time went on, things started to change as now after sitting and waiting for some movement I then found the opposite, I now was experiencing diarrhoea. How could this be I asked myself ? but thought "strange", but nothing of it. Weeks went by and I found myself losing weight and noticed that every time I ate food I would experience a strong pain in my stomach and the urge to run to the toilet. Now the constipation had stopped and each time I sat on the toilet I was suffering from a lot of diarrhoea. On a daily basis I found that I needed to visit the toilet up to 8 times or more a day before I felt better.

This situation was now becoming my daily routine and the weight was dropping off me. Since this started I had lost around half a stone within a few months and my family were getting very concerned about me. I started to think, well if I don't eat there will be no pain and fewer toilet visits. The reality was I was still suffering regardless. It was time to see my doctor. Deep down I knew something was wrong I felt within myself that it was serious but kept hoping it would go away. I was never sick as a child or even as a teenager, I guess that's why I knew this was not normal. At my doctors first visit he asked several questions and took some blood to be tested. Nothing came back abnormal and his next thought was, could it be a "thyroid" problem. Again tests came back negative. Was it all in my head and was I becoming a hypochondriac ?

Still time passed and no change. Now it was affecting my everyday life. Our son Daniel was now 3 years old and found it difficult to look after him due to the amount of time spent on the toilet as I could be sitting there for up to 30 minutes or more. I was also managing our own business while Jason was working his full time job. Family and friends were starting to think that I had an eating disorder as I was eating very little and was always going to the toilet soon after each meal, the "classic" signs of an eating disorder. I found I was having to justify to everyone that I didn't have an eating problem and after time they finally seemed to understand that there was something wrong with me and not an eating disorder. This intern meant I was receiving the support I needed from my family and friends to help me find out what was wrong with me. I no longer felt I had to hide or justify everything I did.

Dealing with this every day became very draining and my energy levels dropped dramatically. I found dealing with Daniel difficult as I could not keep up with his needs. Shopping was a nightmare as I had to cope with both a 3 year old, shopping and no energy. It became so bad that I tended not to leave the house as I was also scared of not getting to a toilet on time and then having to deal with that situation as well as everything else.

With everyone's concern growing I visited the doctor again as I knew there was something wrong and needed to get to the bottom of it (no pun intended). It's now October 1994 and again my doctor could find nothing wrong. A few days later on a Saturday morning, I noticed a lump next to my back passage. I asked my husband to have a look for me and he told me that there was in fact a lump there. I was feeling sick and had a fever, so we went to our local medical clinic and after seeing the doctor there it was recommended I go straight to hospital. On arrival to the hospitals accident and emergency department, I was seen by a student doctor who after listening to all my symptoms, he came up with the theory that I could have Crohn's disease. This was simply due to the fact that he had only weeks before, been studying what Crohn's disease is and the symptoms associated with it. The lump that I went in for was in fact an abscess, which are also tell tale signs of Crohn's disease. My husband and I were then told that if it was Crohn's, that little is known about how and why you get Crohn's and there is currently no cure. It is known to effect males and females primarily between the ages of 16 -30. We were also told that many sufferers can be in and out of hospital requiring many operations throughout their life. I was then booked in for a barium meal test on the Monday which required drinking a cup full of chalk like substance that is a dye to show inflammation of the bowel area.

So here we were, a Saturday afternoon unsure what was wrong with me and what it all meant. Our drive home from the hospital was a quiet one. What to say and make of what the doctor had told us was very overwhelming. Was I going to die, I'm too young for this, I'm a good person, so why me ? Next we were off to pick up Daniel and how do you tell your parents you may have an incurable disease with little known about it and not understanding it yourself. What a situation to be in. So I did my best to tell them with the help of Jason what it all meant.

Monday morning couldn't come soon enough. When the time finally arrived, I went to the hospital with my father as Jason was at work. After the test I remember the nurse telling me she thought is was Crohn's and that an appointment had been made to see the specialist Dr Paul Pavli in a weeks time. I burst out in tears when seeing my dad and told him what the nurse had said, thank god he was there for me. So again believing I had Crohn's, not knowing anything about it, but the fact there is no cure left us both very worried and concerned. How do I tell Jason that our worse fears have come true ?

Finally the appointment time came and Jason and I met with Dr Pavli. He confirmed with us that it was Crohn's disease and he explained to us in laymen terms that Crohn's is where your immune system thinks your body has an infection and turns itself on to fight the infection. The result is your immune system eating away (in my case) parts of my small bowel tissue resulting in parts becoming diseased and possibly requiring removing via operations. There little known about Crohn's and it's kind of like cancer where it can turn it's self on and off at any time with no warning. There are drugs available that have shown, can help some patients, but for the most part it is trial and error as different patients react differently to each drug. He told me that based on what he has seen to date and current studies that I could expect a possible operation within the next 5 years. I was told at the time I was one of about 200,000 people in Australia that had Crohn's disease. Little was known back then and really today little is still known about the disease. Far more people are being diagnosed today than ever before. The next step was for me to have a colonoscopy, which is to have a mini camera inserted up your back passage and through into the small and large bowel to see if any parts are diseased and if Crohn's was currently active. This test was booked for a few weeks time, so in the meantime, my mother found information on Crohn's for me to read up about. I found this information overwhelming which left me numb and I thought this can't be happening to me. Those weeks before the test were long and draining. I tried to put it all in the back of my mind and pretended that this was not happening, in other words suffering from denial.

The day of the colonoscopy was almost here and so I had to prep myself as your bowel has to be empty for this procedure. I had to drink a litre of horrible tasting liquid, which I can only describe as a salt water taste. It made me want to vomit and caused me more diarrhoea, great, just what I needed. We happened to be at a family dinner that night so while they all ate, I sat on the toilet enjoying the night by myself!! After a long night of toilet visits, the day came and Jason took me in. I was put to sleep and after waking up met with the nurse asking me to drink and eat something. Within minutes I was in immense pain and given pain relief. Next thing I woke up in a hospital ward not knowing what was happening with Jason by my side. My first question was "is Daniel okay", "yes he is with family". I later found out that the colonoscopy confirmed that my Crohn's was active and I had developed a stricture/blockage within my small bowel. I also needed the abscess draining to make matters worse. This was the start of my Crohns journey of many operations and hospital visits that required a massive change to my lifestyle. I could not have ever imagined what I was about to go through over the next 12 years of my life.

Chapter Two – Living with Crohn's

Every day with Crohn's is different. My biggest challenge is that due to the high number of abscesses I have had drained, my rectum muscles have weakened to the point where it is very difficult to hold a bowel motion back for any more than a minute or two. Doctors describe this situation as "being incontinent". As a result I have had many accidents over the years which are very embarrassing and degrading to say the least. These situations are extremely stressful and hard to cope with. Here I am a grown woman who "poos" her pants!! Considering I was toilet trained at a very early age !! Just think about that for a minute, how would you cope with this on a daily basis ?

I regularly find myself sitting on the toilet between 5 to 13 times a day which consists of diarrhoea every time. This takes its toll on me as it becomes very draining to say the least. I become lethargic, dehydrated and my back passage gets very sore. To the point where it becomes so inflamed, the skin cracks, bleeds and each time I go becomes even more painful. The stinging pain can be so unbearable at times that I have asked Jason to blow on my butt to try and relieve   the stinging. The only other way is to use a nappy rash cream, however the down side is that every time I go to the toilet I have to re-apply the cream.

I have good days and bad days. A bad day means I stay at home as I'm spending so much time in the toilet with no energy. A good day means only a few visits to the toilet. These are the days I get to live my life, so I get myself ready to go out and do things that I want to do as well as things that I need to do, such as food shopping, errands, that sort of thing. As I can't work anymore due to my unreliability, I do what I can when I can.

As I still wanted to work in someway, we decided to open a small home salon at the back of our home in Australia. We set it up nicely had it all approved and it got so busy I had to employ a part time hairdresser. Things went great for a while. Then a bad day turned into a bad week, which turned into a bad month. I was not able to keep my current bookings as I was spending a large part of the day in and out of the toilet. I then had to scale the salon down with only a few clients per day. Things didn't get any better and finally I had no option but to close the salon down as I could not be reliable enough for my clients. This crushed me as I loved being a hairdresser and running my salon from home. For me it was the best of both worlds, earning an income and being there for my son as he was growing up.

I do miss being in the workforce and the socialising that goes with it. The people you meet, the friends that you make and the feeling of achievement. As a hairdresser, I got all these things and more and to then not be able to do this anymore was upsetting for me. So now I have to rely on Jason for everything and feel in many ways I have lost my independence. This does play on my mind, however you have to make the best of every situation.

As work now became out of the question we thought about having a second child. The idea grew and Jason and I got quite excited about it.

We did have some concerns on how my illness would affect me being pregnant. But we had Daniel and everything went OK, so did I have Crohn's back then ? and does that mean I should be OK for a second child ? So we made an appointment with the doctor to see what he thought. The news was not good, he recommended not to have any more children for two main reasons;

1) With the amount of time I was spending in hospital was it fair to put another child through that and do I have the ability to look after two children with the amount of time I spend on the toilet.

2) As my Crohn's was very active and little was known back then what complications and possible defects could occur during my pregnancy. The high levels of medication were also a huge concern as it may result in down syndrome.

This was a big shock for us both and I was devastated because I so wanted to have another child. So based on the advice given and all the unknowns we decided not to have any more children. So Jason took action and underwent a vasectomy. In hindsight, it was the best decision to make considering the events that have unfolded with my Crohn's disease over the past years. Luckily we are a very tight family unit and spend lots of time together which helps to suppress the desires for another child.

When I'm out of the house, say doing the food shopping, many times I have to leave my shopping basket and run to the toilet. Thank god all supermarkets in England have toilet facilities (back in Australia no supermarkets had public toilets). Without them, I would not even be able to do such a simply thing as food shopping without the risk of having an accident. Most times I try and take someone with me or what should take a normal person an hour can take me several hours. Did you know that the store temperature plays an important part for me, as the cold has an instant reaction and this causes me to have to literally run to a toilet. So going down the "cold" isles can be a pain in the backside for me. (no pun intended)

Close to my home is a large shopping centre which I frequently visit. I know where all the toilets are which gives me comfort for when the need arises. On one occasion, I felt great, so I wore my nice white trousers, parked the car, then started walking towards the centre. Within a second I felt my stomach turn and thought "PLEASE !! not now" and all but ran to the nearest toilet. Unfortunately I didn't get there in time and had an accident in my nice white trousers. Once I got to the toilet I had to take my pants off and clean up the mess the best I could. I was wearing a wide red belt and had a large handbag. So here I am, wet pants with a brown stain and feeling very embarrassed. How do I get back to the car without anyone noticing ? I put my wide belt low down to cover my backside and I held my handbag behind me. I walked very quickly back to the car and drove home. Luckily I only live a few minutes from the shopping centre. What started out as a good morning turned into a bad afternoon. That was one of many similar shopping centre experiences I have encountered over the years. I normally have a spare change of clothes in my car for these situations, however not this time !! I also carry plastic bags in the car to put on my seat and again, not this time.

Wherever I go, I firstly find out where the toilets are situated. When we plan a trip anywhere we make sure we drive on the roads that have service stops. When booking a train or plane ticket I ask for a seat near to a toilet. My life revolves around the toilet. My husband jokes about buying me a "portapottie" for my birthday. Not such a bad idea in reality !! I might write off to the toilet paper companies asking if they do bulk discounts, I would hate to think of the amount of money I spend on toilet paper each year. I should at this point apologize to all the trees that have been cut down on my behalf.

My worst memory was a few years ago when we were with a group of friends and we visited a seaside town of Brighton in England. It was a very cold day below zero. We had just finished lunch, I had already been to the toilet once in the restaurant, paid the bill, jackets on and then all of a sudden, it just gushed out, down my leg and I ran to the toilet, it was like water !! I was a complete mess. I had to wash my whole jeans in the sink and ended up throwing my underwear away. Once I had cleaned the mess the best I could, I composed myself as I was nearly in tears. I was left with wet jeans to walk back to the car with the temperature below zero. This was one occasion I didn't take a spare set of clothes and no shops were open. We hadn't even had a chance to sightsee yet. So the day was ruined, back in the car for a 30 minute drive so I could shower and clean up properly. I felt so upset for the rest of our friends as we had to leave on my account. They all understood my dilemma and we made the best of a bad situation. I can laugh about it now, but at the time it's the worst feeling in the world, I was so humiliated.

A person without a bowel condition never has to think about possible consequences of just leaving your home or going on holiday. As I mentioned above these times require a lot of thought and in some cases I can't do an activity or travel a certain way. For example, I can never snow ski imagine me cold and at the top of a mountain and needing the toilet. I can't go on a boat trip unless there is a toilet on board. Swimming can also be a challenge depending on how cold the water is and again how far from a toilet I am. When travelling on a plane, I need an isle seat close to a toilet. I'm better to travel business class due to the low number of people per toilet, however the cost involved in this is never really possible.

As a female, I have found many times I have to queue to use a toilet, yet the male toilets never seem to have any queues. It's very difficult to try to explain to others why I need to jump the queue and knowing that I need to get there very quickly. So in many instances, I have had to use the men's or find a disabled toilet. I find a large number of public toilets are very smelly and unclean, but I have no choice, but to use them. As a result, I have developed very strong leg muscles.

Since joining the NACC, the National Association of Crohn's and Colitis, I found being a member is well worth while. I firstly joined when we were back in Australia then joined here in the UK. With membership comes a "Can't Wait Card" This is a card that explains the urgency to use a toilet. I have found that after showing this card, shops who would not normally allow you to use their facilities tend to have more compassion and allow me the use of them. This card has got me out of some potentially disastrous situations over the years and I fully recommend Crohn's sufferers joining. You also receive newsletters with articles, information etc.

You will realise how important your friends are when they have to be very patient with your situation. I remember when nine of us went to New York. It was a "girls" weekend, we planned to do lots of sightseeing and shopping. As we walked around New York, I had to tell the girls on many occasions "keep walking and I'll catch up with you". They all knew what I meant and a few girls would always wait with me. I do remember one time I had to sit down as I needed to go again and felt I had no time. One of my friends, Ange literally ran around to find the closest toilet, then ran back to me grabbed my arm and off we went. I made it in the nick of time thanks to Ange. Without her I know I would have had an accident and that would have ruined my day. True friends will always understand and support you in your time of need or in my case many times of need. My trip to New York was a very big step for me as I was way out of my comfort zone and had no idea where the toilets were located on a daily basis. This did cause stress for me. I was so close to saying "no" to going, but I promised myself that this illness was not going to get in the way of this trip and I need to live my life.

At this point I feel it important to say "thank you" to my family as they also have to live with my illness . By this I mean both sets of parents and John and Paul, my aunt and uncle. It was these two who looked after Daniel during the times I was in hospital in the early days. Jason would drop him off early morning and pick him up late after noon. Without them we would never have made it through. Other times it was our parents who wrote out a roster of when and where they were needed. Family really comes into its own during these times and our words can't thank them enough.

Having Crohn's for me, means I have to watch my diet as I have a low tolerance to certain food groups. I have had to learn over the years what works for me and what doesn't. For example, I can't eat "high fibre" as this will make me go the toilet even more and I think I go enough as it is !! So I try and keep to foods that many would consider are not that healthy. For example I would eat white bread instead of brown bread. Soft foods are generally better for me like mash potatoes over baked potatoes. I love fruit, but again my system cannot cope with too much. Red meat plays havoc with my digestive system. I will get cramps within minutes and can then spend the next few hours in pain and discomfort so I stick to white meats. I definitely can't eat spicy foods, as they go straight through me !! I need to consider the amount of carbohydrates I take in as they also react badly with me. Dairy foods can be too rich so these have to be taken in moderation.

So I have had to learn how to balance what food I eat each day. I still find thirteen years later what works one day may not work the next. If I'm having a flare up, I tend not to eat and keep up with my fluids. Whatever I do eat never stays in my system for very long, as having three bowel resections means the food will pass through my system a lot faster as I now have less bowel than the average person. I can only tolerate small amounts of food, so I tend to eat small amounts more frequently. I feel better when I don't eat because the less I eat, the less time I spend in the toilet. However in the real world, you have to eat in order to live.

If I have a long drive ahead of me I tend not to eat until I arrive, otherwise, a trip that takes one hour can take me three hours due to the number of times I have to stop. This strategy normally works for me, however at times, even with no food in my system, I still have to stop and use the toilet.

Over the years I have tried numerous medications, I am always willing to try just about anything to help me have a normal life. I can't even count the amount of pills that I have taken over the years. I did find that all the steroid drugs came with side effects and some of them made me feel so sick that I couldn't function. I tend to have a very sensitive stomach and the various drugs were making me feel constantly sick and giving me headaches for days at a time. Things were bad enough with the constant diarrhoea and cramps in my stomach, so the added side effects from these drugs were pushing me to the limit.

A few years ago I was told I had developed Osteoporosis, "great news" !!! Another challenge to deal with !! This was due to the large amounts of medication my body has endured over the years resulting in my bones becoming weaker. Now I have to take calcium tablets each day to keep it in check.

Steroid type drugs are said to be the best choice to suppress the immune system which can reduce and control a Crohn's flare up. I was also on various types of pain relief. For me however this all came at a price. The side effects I encountered were;

- Mood swings, happy on minute, crying the next
- Forgetfulness of days and dates
- Vagueness of past events

- Fluid retention
- Loss of taste
- Hallucinations
- Sickness
- Loss of hair
- Tooth decay

As a result I felt I had two choices. (1) to keep taking these prescribed medications and put up with the side effects or (2) take myself off all these drugs and live one day at a time and in the process giving me a better quality of life. Some information I was reading suggested no matter how much medication you take, if you are going to get a flare up, there is no stopping it.

It was at this point Jason and I spoke about what to do and we decided to give the "medication free" approach a go and see where it took me. I made an appointment to see my then specialist in Australia, Dr Pavli to discuss my decision. He understood my reasons as he's seen first hand what I'm like while on these medications. However he disagreed from a medical perspective and although I understood this I was very determined to follow through and see how things went. My thoughts were, if I get a flare up I will deal with it and take whatever medication is required at the time to get it under control. Once under control, I would go back to my "medication free" approach. Dr Pavli had never before had a patient like me, stubborn, strong willed and very determined.

I knew in order for this approach to work I had to remain very positive, upbeat and tackle each Crohn's challenge head on. As time went on I found this approach was working for me. When I had a flare up I dealt with it the best I could until I could no longer cope at home and took myself into hospital for the required medical treatment.

When we moved to Manchester UK I was very scared as to who was going to treat me. I had built up such a great trusting relationship with Dr Pavli and was concerned as to who my new specialist would be and how he/she would view my unorthodox approach. We met with Dr J Crampton and passed on my medical notes from Australia. We also discussed my way of dealing with Crohn's. Right from the start we hit it off, he said, although he had never come across a "no drug" approach, he was very interested to see how it worked. After all, he said you know your body better than anyone. I became a test case for Dr Crampton which was great for me as I had direct access to him and his medical team.

He was impressed with my outlook and positivity as he has seen so many Crohn's sufferers over the years who become depressed and all but give up on themselves. He likes to look at things from a patient's perspective. So we came to an agreement to deal with each flare up on a case by case basis. To date this management of my Crohn's is still working well for me. Even though I have had a huge amount of operations and hospital stays, my quality of life is far more important to me than constantly popping pills everyday and rattling as I walk.

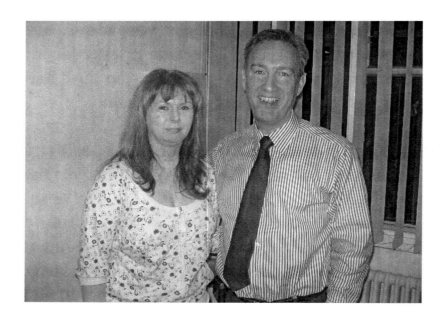

This is me just after a bowel resection operation
with my specialist Dr JR Crampton

Never be scared to question what a doctor tells you. Listen to your body as you will find your "gut feeling" is generally correct. What works for one person may not work for others. Staying strong and positive is key to controlling your illness. You can either allow it to control you or you can control it. It's as simple as making a decision and not compromising no matter what challenges are thrown in front of you.

So many times I wake up and think why me, what have I done to deserve this ?? How much more can I possibly take, I just want to die. Even when I'm at my lowest point, I always find the strength to carry on, I dig deep within myself and I build myself back up into a positive state. You only have one chance at life, so don't waste it by feeling sorry for yourself and giving up. This is the way I live my life and I'm proud of how I have coped. If I can do it you can as well.

Living with Crohn's is hard enough, I don't think I would have made it so far without the love and support of my husband Jason. When it comes to the wedding vows we said to each other many

years ago, "in sickness and in health", by god
Jason has lived up to his part of those marriage
vows. His care for me, I think goes beyond the call
of duty. For example, how many husbands would
blow on their wives butt to help relieve the pain ??

A very important part of living with Crohn's is the
aftercare that's required once I get home from
hospital. This is when Jason's support and help
comes into play. There are so many examples I
could share as to what he does for me so rather
than bore you with them all, here are just a few.
When I arrive home after having an abscess
drained, I normally have a deep cut that requires
daily packing with gauze and solution. Remember
the location of these cuts are always just next to
my anus. So each day Jason has to remove the old
dressing, clean up the cut and pack it with a new
dressing.

I remember once while we were away from home
I became very sore around my bottom, so Jason
had to look and see what was wrong. He found an
abscess had formed and was full of pus. We called
the hospital and was advised to pop the outer area

and remove the pus as soon as possible. This was to prevent the abscess popping on the inside as this can lead to septicaemia which can cause death within hours if not treated. So Jason then had to play doctor and drain the pus from the abscess then drive me to the nearest hospital, so not the fun holiday I was expecting.

With any major operation, when I get home I am still very weak so Jason has to do everything for me. I can't shower on my own, dry or dress myself. So as you can understand there is a lot for him to do which he does without complaining, showing any signs of anger or resentment towards me. In my eyes this is true love and commitment. He always has a way of boosting me up when I'm down, he knows just what to say and do when I need it the most. So if there was a "husband of the year award" Jason would get my vote every year.

Chapter Three – Operations/Hospital stays

To date I have had 50 operations, of which none have been easy. You never get used to it and the fear you feel is always with you, hospitals are a scary place but at times can be the only place you need to be. I remember my first operation as if it was yesterday, I was feeling scared and nervous, sometimes I think I may not wake up and have to say goodbye just in case. In fact some years ago I wrote a letter to my husband and son expressing my feelings and thoughts just in case I don't wake up ! Its natural to feel and think this way, but hey, I'm still here alive and kicking. I have included this letter at the end of this chapter to help others understand my state of mind.

Most of my operations except 3 have been perrianal abscesses, this is a very painful swelling filled with pus that is located next to my back passage. These are caused from the amount of diarrhoea I have on a daily basis. They need to be drained fairly quickly, because if they burst, you

45

can get septicaemia and become very sick to the point where it becomes life threatening.

When I have an abscess I feel sick and usually have a fever, I feel very sore and find it hard to sit down. This means I need to go to hospital. The operation is very quick but is also painful afterwards. They put you to sleep and drain the abscess and in most cases pack the hole with gauze which later the nurses change. A few days in hospital then you can go home.

Once home there is still a lot of maintenance involved for the cut to heal. When living in Australia a local nurse would visit the house each morning to change the dressing. This went on for about a week or so and after that time, it was left to my husband Jason to change the dressing until the wound closed up. With this type of operation it is not possible to stitch up the cut and it needs to close and heal by way of packing the cut and covering it with dressings. When we moved to England, the process for the operation was the same, however packing the dressing each day once I left hospital was left up to us. We could call a doctor to our home if required.

For me a few weeks later another abscess would build up, and back again I would go, this was my life over an 8 year period. In fact it got to the point where I should have been given my own car parking space. I even started knowing all the names of the nurses and doctors in the accident and emergency department. When Jason and I would arrive it was a case of "Hi Mel, back again" ?? it was a bit like my "home from home" Knowing everyone did seem to work in my favour as I would get seen quicker.

Around 2001, I remember having another abscess drained. This was number 45 and thinking will this ever end ?. So… back to hospital I go. As you can imagine I was getting fed up with this whole abscess "thing" and felt very angry that it kept happening to me. I would ask myself over and over what have I done to deserve this ?? My emotions where high at this point and I started to feel depressed. How many more of these can I take ??

Once admitted and taken up to the ward, I spoke with my surgeon.

He showed me an x-ray of the abscess and the area around it and said he thinks he may be able to stop them re-occurring. Great news I thought, but decided not to get my hopes up too much as I had heard this before. Has he really found a way of stopping them ?? Off to theatre I went with a positive outlook, did my usual goodbyes and hoped for the best.

After the operation I awoke in the recovery room and Mr Wilson, my surgeon came to see me and told me "success, I believe I have found the track that allows them to keep returning and building up". He did say that time will tell, but was very optimistic.

Mr Wilson is my 3rd and current surgeon since being diagnosed with Crohn's. He is the only one to have found the "track" and stop these horrible abscesses from returning. However there is no guarantee that they won't come back, so all I can do is live in hope they don't return.

Here are a two suggestions that I used to help ease the pain after these operations.

1) I would fill a large plastic bowl with ice and sit in it for about 5 to 10 minutes. This would numb the area enough to give me relief from the pain and I did this 3 to 4 times a day.

2) Buy yourself an air filled "donut ring". I bought mine from a chemist/drug store. For about the first week or so, I found it very difficult to sit down on any chair. The "donut ring" is fantastic as when you sit on it, it removes any pressure from the wound and gives you comfort and allows you to sit down.

Before I talk about my other operations I want to share with you one particular experience I will never forget. Once again I felt an abscess and so we went off to hospital and was taken through A&E into a treatment/assessment room. I remember it was some time and so I told Jason to go home as it was very late in the evening. Just after he left in came a doctor who examined me and agreed I had an abscess and that it needed draining. I prepared myself for the usual process.

He then left and came back after a short time. I thought he was going to take a second look with regards to the size etc of the abscess. The next moment will stay with me forever. I felt extreme pain as he put a needle straight into the abscess without any warning or pain relief. I screamed in pain to the point I became hysterical and shouted him to stop, he then just said "I will give you a minute to compose yourself" ?? I grabbed my mobile phone and called Jason. The doctor told me not to use the phone and I told him to just watch me.

I remember not being able to explain to Jason what had happened, I simply could not get my words out. I was so upset with what this doctor had just done. Jason arrived very quickly and calmed me down enough to explain what had happened. He was very angry and demanded to speak with the doctors supervisor. He also told the doctor not to come back in the room. His supervisor arrived and was told what had happened. She then went away and a few minutes later both her and this doctor came back in. He was full of apologies and simply didn't realise what pain he had caused me due to his lack of medical experience. He saw it as a boil or blister and thought he would just pop it with a needle. Little did he know or bother to read my notes that I'm always under a general anaesthetic for an abscess drainage.

The other 3 operations I have had were bowel resections. These were due to strictures between my small and large bowel. These operations are much more complicated and classed as a "major" operation. My first bowel operation was in 1995. In fact it was the first Crohn's related operation for me.

Imagine how I felt, Dr Pavli (my specialist back in Australia) tells me I should expect an operation in around 4 to 5 years time, then I find myself in hospital within months of being diagnosed and being told I need a bowel resection. But I thought it would be years before I should expect such a major operation ?? No one can prepare you for bad situations, or how to deal with them . I wasn't ready for this !! this is not how my life should be !! But the reality was, it is, welcome to Crohn's.

My symptoms were, major abdominal pain to the point where I would have to curl myself into a ball and rock back and forth trying to ease the pain. During this it was coming out both ends at the same time. I was a complete mess !! Diarrhoea one end, throwing up the other. I could not eat as this would intensify the pain. I thought giving birth to my son was far easier than this !! Its hard for people to fully understand this type of pain.

There I was lying down, being prepped for the operation. Everyone was being very nice and reassuring, however this did not help my anxiety. All these tubes and wires stuck to my body then I was asked to count backwards from 10. 10.. 9.... Out like a light !! Many hours later I awoke in the recovery room to see Jason sitting by the bed. What a relief, it's all over. Once I was taken back to the ward and had woken up properly, I noticed I had more tubes and wires than I started with. I didn't want anyone to see me this way, especially my son, what would he think he is only 4 years old.

Both the surgeon and doctor visited me to tell me the outcome of the operation. They had found my Crohn's was very active and removed about 30cm's (12 inches) of my small bowel. I was told that fingers crossed, I would not require an operation like that again for some time, however once you start operating on the bowel, there is a higher chance that you will require further operations later on in life.

I had a new best friend, my pain relief machine. All I had to do was press this button and it gave me pain relief. However I also found it was causing me to throw up. Now this was painful as they used staples instead of stitches for my stomach. I had to put a pillow over my stomach to try and ease the pain.

I was very determined to make a quick recovery, I was told it will be 6 to 8 weeks before I can do anything at all. Well I proved them wrong and was back into the swing of things within 3 to 4 weeks. After being home I noticed the scar left from the operation was huge. I thought it made me look ugly. I didn't want anyone to see the scar and how could I wear a bikini again. I felt very self-conscious to the point I was embarrassed to be naked in front of my husband. In time I did get over this and simply accepted it as part of my life with Crohn's. Jason's feelings towards me had not changed, he had no issues, it was me thinking he did without asking his opinion.

This was the only resection operation while living in Australia. In 2003, 8 years later I found myself in a similar situation which required a second resection. The tests confirmed it was in the same spot as my first. This time there was a possible twist. Depending on what they find and the amount of diseased bowel that requires removing, could mean I would be given a temporary bag. This bag is called a stoma and is attached to the side of my hip and all your body waste is sent via a tube to this bag. I then have to remove and empty the stoma bag when it gets full. The idea is to allow the bowel to rest and heal for about 12 months then the stoma is removed and the bowel is then reconnected, which means another operation !!

Oh my god, a scar is bad enough, but now I could possibly have a bag stuck to my skin. How does anyone cope with this, I was feeling pretty scared I didn't want this, in fact, I didn't want any of this. Can't someone else have my life? But after a deep breath, you get through it, you deal with it and you move on. One thing I have learned is that no matter what I go through, there is always someone worse off than me. In the end I didn't require a stoma this time, and was very thankful for that.

My second resection (2003) was a little easier to cope with as I knew what was ahead. The fears are still there, and you wish none of this was happening. One of my concerns was; are they going to use the same scar, or am I getting another one. I can see it now, my stomach is going to be a picture of noughts and crosses.

They did use the same scar, only this time I had stitches and the scar got longer, and no stoma bag. After a few weeks I was getting back to my old self again, but as you get older it does take a lot out of you. This is where you need lots of patience and a really good book.

Three years later its now 2006, and I am back having more tests, same symptoms and in the same spot. This means another bowel resection, thank god you have lots of bowel. To date I believe around 50 centimetres of my small bowel has been removed. This has been a hard year, in fact the hardest yet. It started at the beginning of the year with me going to hospital with a flare up, I needed another operation, but first we tried to contain the disease with medication and bed rest. That worked for a while, I spent my birthday in hospital which wasn't easy, then went home without having the operation. In July, things got worse and so back into hospital I went. This time I spent my husband's birthday in hospital. It was his 40th and I had planned a big party for him, which had to be cancelled. There's not much you can do about social events etc as my health has to come first. Luckily, my husband wasn't too concerned as he had his own issues about turning 40 and just wanted to sulk in the corner feeling sorry for himself.

This time the medication and rest was not enough and so another operation was needed. My specialist and surgeon wanted to try a different form of pain relief this time so they came up with the idea of an epidural. This is something I have never had before so I was feeling quite anxious. For those who don't know an epidural is where they put a needle and tube in the base of your spine and administer the pain relief to numb you from the waist down. This is commonly used during child birth. Unfortunately for me, they were not able to get the needle into my spine as the gap between my bones was too small. This process was very frightening for me and I was looking forward to this form of pain relief as I do not react well to morphine or similar type of pain relief drugs. So as you can imagine, I then became more nervous knowing what was ahead of me once the operation was over.

As I was taken into theatre, Jason walked with me and stayed until he was asked to leave. This is always something you never get used to, having to say goodbye before an operation as who knows what could happen. You can't help thinking at this time of the long recovery process ahead of you once the operation is over. You feel so helpless afterwards as you are not allowed or in a position to do anything for yourself. So after been given a sedative it was now time for the anaesthetist to put me under for bowel resection number three ! The operation went well and only a small section of my small bowel was removed which meant I escaped without requiring a stoma bag. Once again they were able to cut into my existing scar, which is now increasing in length each time. It's now twenty-one centimetres long. I think after my first operation the scar was about 11 centimetres long.

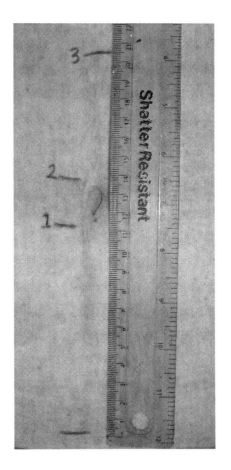

This is a photograph of my scar. As you can see I have marked all 3 bowel resections. The scar now covers most of my stomach area.

This recovery was the hardest to date. I looked and felt like a train wreck. The drugs were really taking their toll on me and I was completely out of it for most of the first week. I don't remember much of it at all only that I was having really scary nightmares and hallucinations to the point where I was frightened to close my eyes. The only time I felt safe to sleep was when Jason was there. As I was weaned off the morphine I began to feel human again and I was on the road to recovery. As each day passed more tubes were taken off me. I had now been in hospital for three weeks and it was time to go home. I normally recover well after a few weeks of being at home. This time however, it was the complete opposite. On arrival home from hospital I found myself throwing up after each meal. Now that is quite normal for me as it takes up to a week for my stomach to tolerate food again.

Two weeks later I was still throwing up so back to hospital. At first it was thought it could be a blockage caused by the operation. As a result of this I was admitted back in and was not allowed to eat. Due to me throwing up so much I became dehydrated, just another issue to deal with !!! My normal specialist was away on holiday at this time and so I was put under another specialist. She made me feel very uncomfortable due to her poor bedside manner and her lack of interest and understanding as to what I had to say. I know my own body better then anyone can !! After a few days rest things started to move and I was discharged.

Still not feeling 100% well, a few weeks later, I needed to get out of the house to avoid going stir crazy, we decided to go to the cinema
to see a movie. It was great to finally get out and the movie was good. On leaving the cinema, I started to feel strong stomach cramps, these came in waves every few minutes. They increased in strength (I would describe them just like labour pains) and I started to double over with the pain. I just needed to get home ! Within the hour of being home, I was in terrible pain, throwing up, I couldn't move. Jason called for an ambulance I was screaming in pain by now. When the ambulance crew arrived I was taken straight back to hospital. After an x-ray, the surgery team were

put on notice that they may need to operate. A few hours later it was suggested my bowel had looped due to the recent operation. I was not healing as I should have and it was now a waiting game as to the next course of action. It was decided not to operate again and that more hospital rest was needed. I was in for about a week before allowed to go home.

I had lost a lot of weight and was very weak. I was thinking, will this year ever end !! As the weeks passed I started to improve and months later I am happy to say I feel great. I can only hope that I can now have a good few long years without any more problems, god knows I deserve a break.

Throughout the last thirteen years in between operations, I have required over 100 hospital stays, which were caused by a flare up of the Crohn's disease. These flare ups required bed rest, no eating and medication which is given intravenously. This means the drugs are given through your veins. Generally, I am given a heavy course of steroids to help suppress my immune system allowing the flare up to calm down and my body returning to normal. Normally my bowel works over time and so this slows down any movement giving me the rest I require.

These stays are normally around one to two weeks depending on how severe the flare up is. Each stay means needles, x-rays, blood tests, scans and toilet visits !! I strongly suggest you bring your own toilet paper and baby wipes. I also recommend you do whatever it takes to get yourself a private room as there is nothing worse than needing the toilet and having to wait because I have very little time between needing to and actually going.

Every time I go to hospital, I have to face one of my biggest fears, that being a canular needle. This is a needle that is placed into my vein to allow fluids and medication to pass intravenously. When I am "nil by mouth" meaning I am not allowed to eat or drink anything, this is the only way they can keep me hydrated and when the drugs are administered this way they take immediate effect.

Over the years my veins have started collapsing which has meant the doctors find it very difficult to find a vein that will sustain the canular. This process is very painful as it's like someone stabbing you in the arm over and over again until they find one. Years ago it would only take one or two tries which I could deal with. As time passed the number of attempts to find a suitable vein dramatically increased. It got to the point where I could not cope and I would do anything to avoid going into hospital. I remember at times waiting up to a week hoping my symptoms would subside so I would avoid going to hospital and enduring the canular needle.

My worst memory was back in Australia when the doctor tried 14 times to find a vein. My arms were black and blue with bruises, I was crying and telling him to stop. The only reason he stopped was because my husband all but grabbed the doctor and told him if he tried again he would knock him out and that no one should undergo that sort of treatment. The average tries to find a suitable vein is around 5 to 6. My arms are that bad that the doctors now resort to my feet and neck. Worst case is when they place a central line into my chest. There is also the matter of taking blood. This is done each day and cannot be taken from the canular. So as you can now imagine, I again become a pin cushion. They have even had to take blood from my groin area and that has to be one of the most painful things I have experienced and would not want this to happen again. In fact the last time I had blood taken was when I saw my specialist as an "out patient". I walked out of the clinic with 8 to 10 plasters on both arms. Those waiting to have blood taken all looked at me and I said "you would think they would know how to take blood by now !" and walked out.

You can't prepare a child to see their own mother in a hospital bed attached to monitors with tubes and leads everywhere. So Jason and I took the decision not to let Daniel see me until most of the tubes etc were gone and the swelling reduced. When he did visit I normally still had a canular hooked up via a machine which administered the drugs at the correct dosage. This machine is on wheels so I can still walk around. Daniel would always ask what this machine did, so after explaining it's purpose, over time he started calling it "Barney". So in a way he was happy to see "Barney" helping his mum get better. The name "Barney" is still used today which gives us all a giggle.

When I had my last major operation, Daniel was now 16 years of age and he asked if he could see me straight after the operation which we agreed to. I had only just got back to the ward and I was still waking up when he arrived with Jason. I still don't remember this and have to rely on what they told me happened. Daniel was taken back by what he saw and this did upset him and now understands why we wouldn't allow him to see me like this when he was younger.

When I first started having hospital stays I found lots of family and friends would always be visiting me with flowers, cards etc. Their constant support was a real comfort to me as a hospital can be a very lonely place as I'm usually in a ward with elderly patients. Having to spend all day in bed with little to do you crave company from friends and family. I look forward to visiting hours hoping someone will walk through the door.

When we moved to England the hospital stays became more difficult for me as I have less family here and few friends. The days became very long and drawn out, with only Jason and Daniel visiting each day I really cherished the time we had together. Here in England they are very strict on visitors, even with family members, so I only got to spend a few hours a day with them. As time went on, we made friends and it became easier as they started to visit me to show their support and I thank them for that. My mum and dad would always call me from Australia the same time every night to ask how I was feeling and I always looked forward to their call and hearing their voices.

Over the years I have learnt it is very important to take into hospital the comforts from home that work for you. As the hospital does not have the ability to provide you with what you need and are used to. It now only takes me a few minutes to pack what I need as its now second nature. Things like:

- Your own soft toilet paper

- Tissues
- Pillow
- Sheep skin mat for your bed to prevent bed sores.
- Moisturiser
- Lip balm
- Pen and paper
- A cheap watch
- Mints or breath freshener

Always leave any valuables at home as things do tend to go missing, it's sad to say but very true. These are my essential items whenever I am admitted into hospital. I hope this list helps you when considering packing your own bag for hospital.

As I have a real fear of not waking up after surgery, I felt compelled to write a letter to my family in case something did happen to me during an operation. I wanted to leave them both with a few words of how I felt and give them some comfort if the worst did happen. Here is the letter I wrote which I felt was important to include in my book. Although a very personal letter, Jason and Daniel felt it was important to include.

Dear Jason and Daniel,

If you are reading this letter, then I must be now with god in heaven. I will be always watching over you both and I want you to know my life was so complete having you both in it. I have never felt so loved more in my life than from the years I have had with you both. Keep each other safe and take care of yourselves, you need each other now more than ever.

Daniel, I am so proud of you and how you have grown into such a wonderful young man. I have always known that you are going to have all your dreams come true. Your life is going to be filled with much love and happiness. Just know that my love for you will last a life time. Be good for your dad, he needs you now and remember the decisions he makes for you are from love. He only wants the best for you. Goodbye my darling son, having you was the best thing I could have ever wished for. I love you more than words can say. Always remember that. (Always your loving mum xxx)

My Darling Jason, thank you for the best years of my life, you made me the happiest woman in the world. You are the kindest, most generous man I have ever met and I was so proud to be called your wife. You were the best husband to me, the way you always kept me safe, you always took such good care of me when I was sick. We had a wonderful life together, full of love and happiness and what a wonderful son we made. You have so much love inside you, I want you to share it with others and I especially want you to have a happy life, god knows you deserve it. You made me very proud of you, your one in a million.

Don't be sad. Think about all those fun times we shared, didn't we laugh !! Be strong, Daniel needs you now. Life goes on and so must you, fulfil all your dreams, be happy, I want only the best for you. I will always love you, I thanked god everyday for bringing you into my life.

Take care of each other, my love will be with you both forever and always.
Mel
xxx

Chapter Four – Husband and Son's Perspective

In 1988 I married Melanie, what we had to go through to get married was crazy. She is Catholic and I am Presbyterian and Mel wanted to be married in a Catholic Church. I remember well part of our wedding vows, "in sickness and in health". At the time I thought little of it as it's just part of what you say when getting married. I must say that I now really do understand what it means and have been living by those words for many years now.

When we were sat down late 1994 and told my wife had Crohn's, I didn't know what to think as I had no idea as to what it all meant. First I thought OK no problem some emotion, but on the whole naïve really. The time when it did hit me was shortly after that when Mel was kept in hospital after having the colonoscopy test (basically they put a tiny camera up your butt and look around the large and small bowel). I arrived to pick her up to be told, that she needed to be admitted from the results of the test. OK I thought, better to be safe then sorry as they say (all the time still not knowing or understanding what was going on and why). The emotion I felt is very hard to put into words and a very strong feeling of helplessness. I guess I'm one of these husbands that likes to think he is a super hero, always there to protect my wife and family. But in this case having no control and no understanding was very disconcerting to say the least.

All I could do was sit by and support Mel every step of the way. At the time I did not realise that was just what Mel needed and it meant so much to her. You soon realise how much we think about ourselves and not other people every day of our lives. Here I am focusing on how I felt, thoughts about me me me, while all this time here is my wife lying in a hospital bed with no idea what was going on and in need of my support to reassure her I was there to watch over her. Sitting there for hours on end just watching her while she sleeps in hospital gave me time to think and I came up with a plan on how I would deal with Crohn's as a husband.

Crohn's is a disease that effects the whole family and although I don't physically go through the operations, hospital stays, the day to day pains and visits to the toilet that Mel does, I still go through all the emotions and concerns that this terrible disease brings. So my plan was simple; keep positive, be realistic, never just except what doctors have to say at face value, be on guard, ask good questions and don't stop until you understand or get the answers you are wanting. For me my part of this marriage in these times was to be the watch dog for Mel's better health and in times to come, her sanity.

At the time of being told Mel had Crohn's we were both still very young, I was early twenties, married, a child and a wife with a disease that still to this day has no cure or much understanding. But those wedding vows came flooding back and I was committed to always being there no matter what was thrown at us. I looked into what was known about Crohn's and although found medical information, I was not able to find anything that could help me as a husband/partner of a Crohn's sufferer. For me to write this chapter,

I hope will help all those partners understand and give a positive spin on what is a terrible illness.

It's funny when I think back over the years and remember whenever people talk to us both about Mel's Crohn's, they always seem to pity her and feel sorry for what she goes through, when she has her hospital stays again similar things happen. Of course this is normal and to be expected, however during these times I found few people would ever ask how I was coping. Thankfully my parents and Mel's parents would always ask this question as they, at times were very much in the "front line". I found this support priceless and much needed. As a partner be ready for this and remain positive and just get on with it. Your life will change and you will find it hard to cook, clean, look after the family, go to work, visit the hospital everyday etc etc etc. There are always jobs that need doing, so you need to be well organised and disciplined if you are going to cope. Life can't stop, bills still need to be paid and your responsibilities don't simply stop because your wife is in hospital.

I had to rely on family in order to be able to continue working, have Daniel looked after and visit Mel. When Mel was in hospital for the first time I was working as a news cameraman for a television station which meant shifts and at times trips for up to six weeks at a time as my main role involved politics and tracking the Prime Minster of Australia. So I organised to work only day shifts when ever Mel was in hospital. A few years later I was given an opportunity to change my career. If I worked hard in a short time I would be able to have the time to look after both Mel and Daniel while still making a good income so I took the chance, and changed my career.

This change has made coping with hospital stays a lot easier as I now have the time I need to get everything done whilst still having time to see Mel in hospital. So I guess I changed my career in order to cope with Mel's illness. Looking at it now it was the best decision I ever made, however back then it was a real "make or break" decision.

Over the years we have developed two modes of living.

1) Hospital mode – While Mel is in hospital
2) Home mode – When Mel is at home.

Each of these modes means certain things and responsibilities. For our son Daniel, while growing up he though it was normal to have these two ways of living and so, was able to adapt. To this day when ever Mel goes into hospital I find myself saying to Daniel, "right mums going into hospital, so it's hospital mode son". I see the three of us as a team and we must work together in order for our lives to work and cope with Crohn's, you won't always get it right, but if you don't give up, you will come out on top every time. I am proud to say that Daniel has grown up into a young adult that we are both very proud of and in many ways Mel's Crohn's situation has played a role in this.

During many of Mel's hospital stays, which to date has hit the 100 mark, I always found it hard to leave because years ago there were no bed side televisions, just a radio if it worked. I would always ask if there were any other Crohn's patients on the ward and many times would overhear conversations between these couples and if possible talk and listen with them and their partners and what I heard and found on many occasions was alarming. Many times I remember it was the boyfriend or husband that seemed very intolerant to the situation and to the point where I witnessed them blaming their partner that they had to come into hospital. How inconvenient it was for them with comments like "the world doesn't stop just because your in hospital" "it's always about you" etc. One time Mel was in hospital we met an older female who had Crohn's and the next time we met was again in hospital and when I asked how her husband was, she told me he had left her as he decided he couldn't cope with her disease and wasn't prepared to live like that. I was speechless and thought to myself I will never let Mel down like that no matter what. It just shows how some people can be, weak, shallow and selfish.

So…. time for you to read about my time in hospital. I like to make myself at home, as you get to know the nurses on the ward, I found I could have a joke and make the best of it. Many times I jump into the bed with Mel and fall asleep and at times kick Mel out on a chair while I lay down for a nap and now days, watch a bit of television. I have no problem asking for things and at times just helping myself. I now bring in a portable DVD player and we lay on the bed together and watch a movie, eat some popcorn and if Mel is feeling OK a little snuggle. The down side is that from time to time the nurses come in !!

The other side is when Mel has just come out from an operation. The first time I saw her there with all these tubes and things all over her was very distressing, but now that I understand what they do and their need, you tend to see past them. My advice is simply to be there for when they wake up. Be the first person they see when they wake up from the operation and even though, they won't remember it at all, I know on a subconscious level they do. Never be afraid to ask questions to the nurses or doctors about anything. Many times I would speak to a doctor or nurse about Mel's state of mind to help them understand how she is feeling. This has always been welcomed by the hospital staff. I must also mention a deal that Mel and I have prior to her going into surgery. I will always go with her when she is taken to the surgery prep room. I will stay with her right up until she is taken into theatre. Mel has a fear that she may not wake up after an operation and so being there means so much to her.

When it's time to take Mel to hospital we always pack her bag which saves me having to then leave her go back home pack some things and return hoping I got everything she needs. It's also important as a partner to know and understand the hospital process. What I mean by this is when you first enter hospital, 95% of the time you have to be admitted through A&E (accident and emergency) This is where you tell them the problem they assess and hopefully within a few hours get to see a doctor. All I can do is sit and listen and help out where I can with some of the questions asked to Mel.

In all cases so far Mel has been admitted which means having a canular or intravenous drip put in her arm. I have to sit and watch as they try time after time to find a vein without success because over the years, due to the high number of canulars,

Mel's veins now keep collapsing or the doctors simply can't find a suitable vein or one at all. One time a doctor tried 14 times, Mel was in tears and I suggested to the doctor he stops before I punch him. His bed side manner needed some work as did his understanding as to the amount of pain Mel was in. I also remember another time where I told the doctor to stop trying the put the canular in and leave the room. I then called in his supervisor which resulted in Mel receiving an apology from this doctor and they finally listened and acted on the fact that Mel has poor veins. So often the doctors ignore us when we tell them the situation of Mel's veins. The unfortunate thing is she needs to have one put in, so it's a case of go until it works. As you can read from above, I am not backward in telling them what I think and if needed, usher them out the room while Mel composers herself.

One real frustrating thing is I know far more about Crohn's and how to treat and deal with it than most nurses and A&E doctors. You see every time we went in it was the same thing. What's wrong, symptoms, history pain level etc. When it comes to Mel's pain relief the only drug she can take is pethidine, now A&E don't like to use this drug due to its addictiveness. I can see them thinking are we hear because Mel is a drug addict looking for a fix ? or she is simply treated as a drug addict until they believe different. Mel needs 100 milligrams and every time they come back with either 25 or 50. I suggest to the staff they read Mel's medical notes and history as it clearly states Mel needs 100 milligrams. This is an example where I need to stand my ground in order to ensure Mel gets what she needs. It's no fun, but I do understand why A&E works this way. So be ready if you have never experienced the A&E process, you will, however learn how to deal with it very quickly.

When I leave the hospital, its normally straight home making a list of what jobs need to be done and getting on with them. Now that there are bed side telephones I can call Mel at anytime, which has made things so much better as communication between us when she is in hospital is vital to her sanity. There is nothing better then being able to call her and speak with her just before she goes to sleep on a night. So here I am looking after the house, my son Daniel, Mel and my work while she is in hospital. However here is the interesting thing, When Mel is back home and recovered, I seem to slip back into "I do these jobs and Mel does those jobs". To the point where I think I couldn't cope doing what I do when I'm in hospital mode. Crazy but true !!

When Mel is at home, I tend to oversee her eating and many times we might go out for dinner and Mel gets carried away with ordering and I say "no" you won't or can't eat that which does not go down well at the time, however after years of this she tends now to listen to me, but not all time and at those times it usually finishes with "I should of listened to you" or "I told you so". I can imagine the frustration Mel goes through with food.

I guess to summarise as a partner to someone who suffers with Crohn's we need to be positive, compassionate, supportive, understanding and realistic. Simple really !!! When I look back over time I don't see the last 20 plus years with Mel as a day to day grind. I don't keep wishing for things to be different, I have excepted the situation and learned to be positive and be the husband that I committed to when we got married back in 1988. I see the future as bright and even if there is never any more advancement into treatment of Crohn's, I know Mel and I will live a happy life and continue to take on the challenges that Crohn's throws at us.

DANIEL'S PERSPECTIVE

I found growing up that my life was split into two sections, normal life and hospital life. My normal life meaning going to school, meeting up with friends, and spending time with my parents. Not really having a care in the world. This all changes when it comes to hospital life, I did find it very hard to cope with everyday life because of how my mum was in hospital for long periods of time.

It felt like I had two different families being juggled between them both, when it was time to go home from school I knew that some days mum or dad couldn't pick me up, so instead my great aunt and uncle picked me up and they became my second mother and father. They would take me to their home, give me dinner and sometimes I would spend the night there because my dad couldn't pick me up due to him being at the hospital with my mum for most of the night or working a late shift. The good thing I suppose about me being so young is that I didn't understand what Crohn's disease was or how it really affected my mum. Because of this I felt that I didn't have to worry as much about her. When I did however visit my mum in hospital it felt like my home away from home, in a funny way, I felt really comfortable there because I was there so much.

I knew all the nurses and doctors and I even made up my own friend barney who was a machine that delivered amounts of drugs to my mum. I would eat many meals there, do my homework and at times curl up on the bed with mum and watch television. Sometimes I remember finding a wheelchair and racing up and down the ward. I would also blow up the rubber gloves and ended up with a large collection at home. Other times it was very boring and I couldn't wait to get home and play with my toys.

When she was at home it was great! I had my mum back to myself again, but there were times outside of hospital which were tough as well. When my mum and I went to the shopping mall and she needed the toilet I always had to go into the women's toilets and it was so embarrassing to go in and wait right outside the toilet door for my mum to finish. But as much as I hated it, it felt normal and second nature to me.

There were some things that I couldn't really do at all with my mum because of how she always needed to be around a toilet or needed to know at all times where the nearest one is. So because of that, we couldn't really go on long walks just the two of us or play football or do any outdoor activities. Probably one of the things I hated most was when we took trips out to theme parks and there was a ride that I was just dying to go on. We would wait in the queue and just before we got to the front, mum needed to go to the toilet, so we had to leave the queue and when she was done, we had to line up again. As I was young I had no patience's at all especially at theme parks and in the end she couldn't go on them anyway because of how the ride would unsettle her stomach and possibly have an accident on the ride. Therefore it was something my dad and I would do. I did however question things like is there anything in this world I could do with both my parents not just one of them, this did make me sad at times.

I was young when my mum was diagnosed with Crohn's, everything that came along with it just felt like every other day. Looking back now I am 18 years old, I do believe that I have had a tough childhood. I did cope and made the best of a bad situation and I believe we all have a strong spirit, determination, and positive outlook within our family. I admire my mum greatly for everything she goes through every day of her life. Even when she is down or in hospital she is always there for me, smiling and keeping positive.

Printed in the United Kingdom by
Lightning Source UK Ltd., Milton Keynes
138707UK00001B/87/P